This Notebook Belongs To:

____

Made in the USA
Monee, IL
07 July 2026

56550199R00069